Potassium Health Secrets Revealed: The Heart Protector

Create an Alkaline Body with Potassium

"Increase the use of potassium and reduce the Risk of heart attack and Stroke."

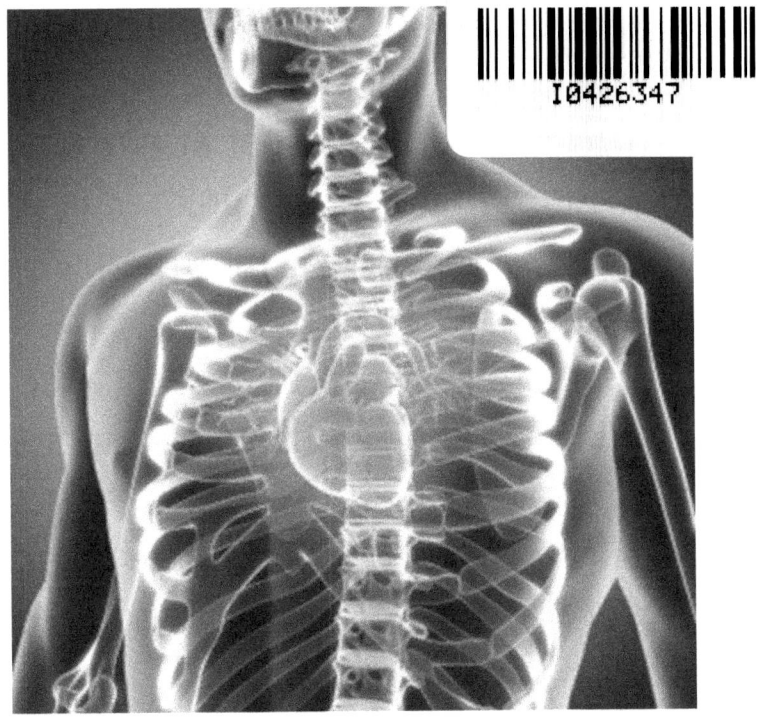

I0426347

By Rudy S Silva, Natural Nutritionist

is not intended for use as a source of legal, business, accounting or financial advice. All readers are advised to seek services of competent professionals in legal, business, accounting, and finance field.

Printed in the United States of America

Table of Contents

Table of Contents..5

1: Introduction 7

2: Potassium and Sodium In Your Body 15

Chapter 3: How Potassium Prevents Diseases 27

4: Foods high in potassium 45

5: Using potassium supplements..........59

About The Author And Other Resources 65

1: Introduction

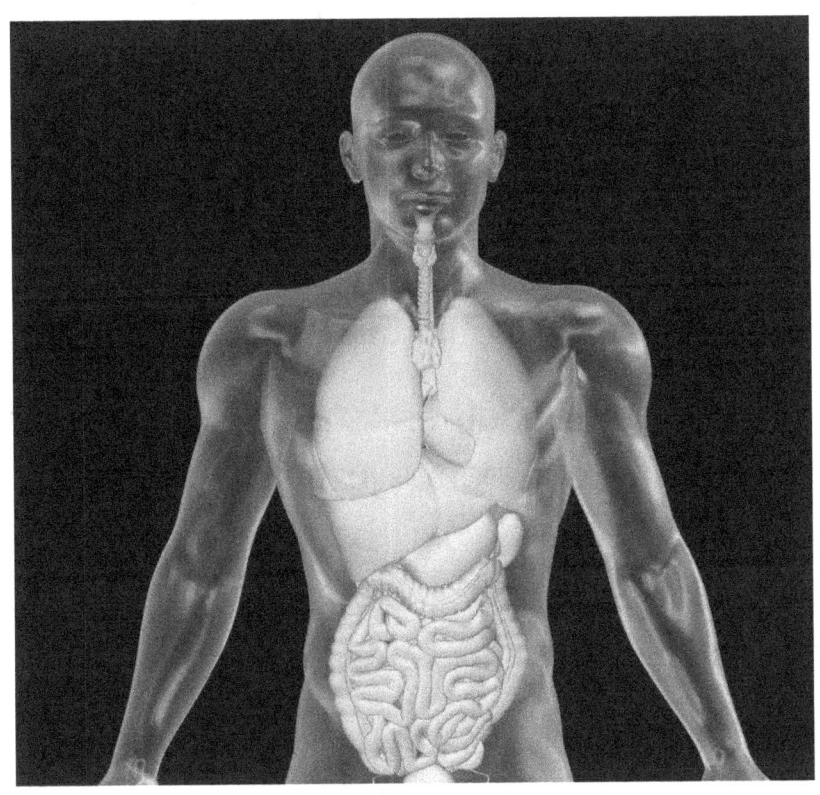

"In Nutrition, Potassium is known as The Great Alkalizer."

Your Heart

Having the right amount of potassium in your body will keep your heart beating. Of course, this is not the only thing that keeps it beating. A good nutritional diet, exercise, a good mental attitude, and with right potassium intake this will ensure a good a healthy heart.

In this e-book, you will learn how and why potassium is used in your body. You will get a list of foods that you need to eat to get potassium and the type of potassium supplement you should take to keep healthy.

Potassium is another mineral that has many activities in your body, just like sodium. As potassium enters your body in food or by supplements, it is transformed into electrical charges called ions.

Potassium and sodium work together to maintain your body at a healthy level. One can't work properly without the other. But potassium does other work that does not require the assistance of sodium. It helps other nutrients to help your muscles and nerves working like they should and to synthesize protein and store carbohydrates.

Potassium Ions

These potassium ions help create electrical potentials across cell membranes and along nerve pathways. What this potential, which is like a battery, does is create a condition where electricity flows where the potential is created by carrying information and nutrients for your cells.

These nutrients that enter your cells come from the food you eat and are burned inside the cells with oxygen to create the energy you need to move around and for all your body functions.

Potassium is an element that is needed and found in all tissues and cells of your body. It helps to provide smooth function and activities for these cells. It is called an intercellular nutrient since is found mostly inside the cell liquid.

Potassium is found in all foods but it's easier to absorb it from vegetables and fruits.

The Great Alkalizer

Potassium is also known as the "Great Alkalizer" since it easily combines with phosphorus, chlorine, and sulfur, which are all acid residue elements. If you have a slight potassium excess in your body, you will have stamina, good body movement, and may have excellent thought processes. Athletes are potassium people because of the precise body movements, speed, and energy they use. Potassium gives them body and brain health.

It is known that plants need potassium in the soil to grow healthy. Potassium protects plants from diseases and germs and it does the same thing in your body. It helps to make your body alkaline and brings in more oxygen into your cells for more protection against germs that like a low oxygen environment. It keeps your blood at a high alkaline level.

Potassium Losses

Your body needs all the potassium you can eat and on occasion, you will need to take a supplement. Any excess potassium that you have will be excreted in your urine. Your kidneys determine how much potassium should be in your body. If your kidneys are weak or diseased, it may excrete too much potassium through your urine or it may maintain too much in your body.

Severe loss of potassium can initiate a heart attack, however, very few people ever reach this condition.

If your body retains too much potassium, then this upsets the balance of minerals in your body. One result is less calcium will be absorbed and used by your body.

If you do any type of athletic training or physical activity, such as running, bike riding, tennis, and other activities, feeling dizzy or faint during your activity can be related to a loss of potassium. This can be avoided by eating foods that give you a good balance of minerals and perhaps having an electrolyte drink before you practice that does not have sugar.

You can lose potassium when you vomit, have diarrhea, use laxatives or diuretics, sweat excessively, or have surgical drainage.

You can also lose or excrete potassium if you take drugs. Here is a list of drugs that cause you to lose potassium.

- Amphotericin, Antifungals
- Antiparkinsonian Medicines
- Aspirin
- Bronchodilators
- Corticosteroids, Prednisone, Prednisolone
- Digitalis
- Diuretics
- Penicillin
- Tetracyclines
- Ulcer medications
- Sedatives
- Antacids
- Anticonvulsants

- Stool softeners
- Cough Cold Remedies

Potassium and Disease

Potassium is the main ion that is inside your cells and sodium is the main ion outside your cells. This is what makes the electrical potential across your cell membrane causing nutrients to move into the cell and toxin to move out.

If you lack potassium, you can easily build it back up with food or supplements. When your body stores of potassium get too low and it is expressed as low blood potassium, this can be a life threating condition.

It is believed by herbalists that people with cysts, tumors, moles, and warts have a deficiency of potassium.

It was discovered by Dr. Gerson, The Gerson Therapy, that all people that have a chronic disease are low in potassium. When an excess of Na+ is in your cells where potassium should dominate, production of body enzymes is decreased. This condition also disturbs the electrical potential across the cells leading to malfunction of cellular activities.

To counteract the lack of potassium drinking plenty of fresh vegetable and fruit juices is what is required. This can also be done with a good source of potassium supplements, but drinking juices provide you with more minerals that you might be lacking.

2: Potassium and Sodium In Your Body

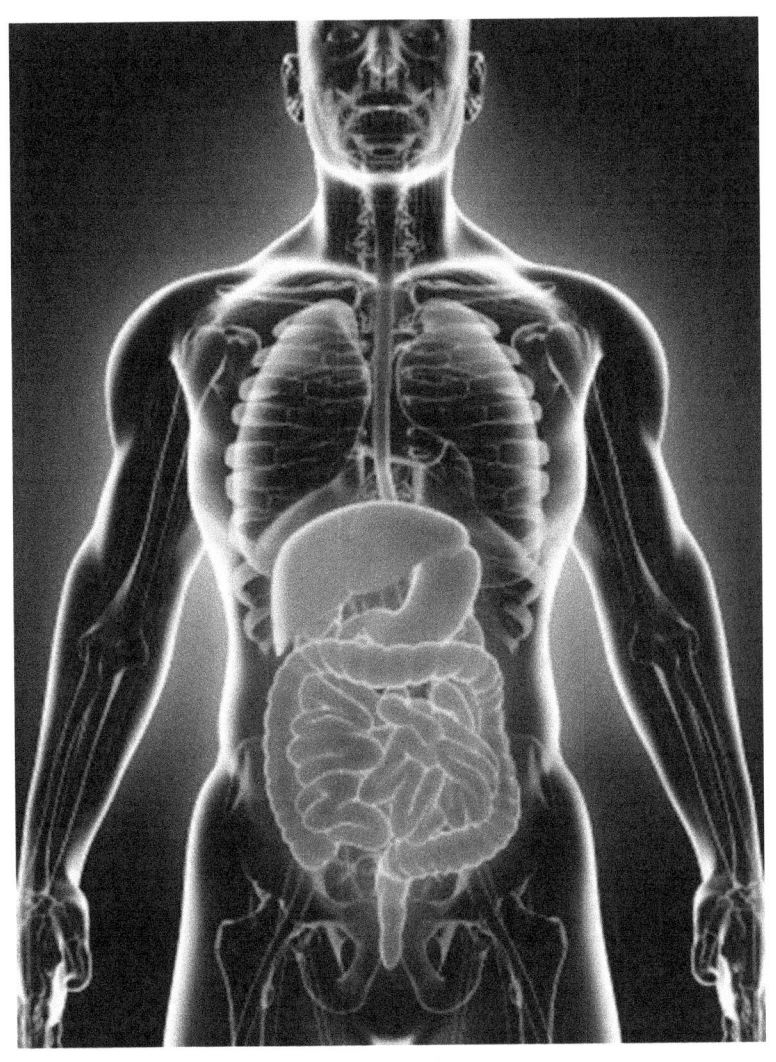

Potassium has a strong influence on the function of the liver and is regulated in your body by iodine.   The real function of iodine is to move potassium and the iodine may have to come from only organic iodine found in natural food to do this.

Since potassium is regulated in the liver, this happens around 2 a.m. in the morning. If you wake up at 2 am in the morning it's an indication that you have an imbalance in potassium. This imbalance most likely will be the use of some medication. Waking up at 3 am in the morning indicates a calcium or magnesium deficiency

The ratio of potassium to sodium in your body is the critical part that has to be maintained so that you have maximum health. Raw foods such as fruits and vegetables have the natural potassium to sodium ratio that needs to be maintained. When you cook this produce, you destroy this ratio and your body finds it hard to recognize this food as good for your body. This affects your well-being and future health.

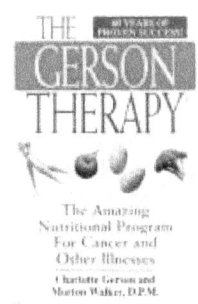

In The Gerson Therapy, 2001, New York, Charlotte Gerson and Morton Walker, D.P.M., point out,

"In his monthly newsletter Health & Healing, Julian Whitaker, M.D. writes, 'The way to bring your sodium-potassium ratio back into balance is to eat lots of vegetables, legumes, whole grains, and fruits. These wholesome foods naturally have an excellent sodium-to-potassium ratio of a least 1:50.' Dr. Whitaker adds that some fruits, such as oranges, offer a good mineral proportion of 1 part sodium to 260 parts potassium."

Potassium and sodium are the main ionic minerals that create the Sodium-Potassium Pump in your cell structure, which allows cells to receive nutrients for cell function and to eliminate toxins and other nutrients from within the cells.

Potassium easily dissolves in water. When it does, it becomes ionized and is an electrically charged molecule. It has one loose electron in its outer orbit and this electron can easily move on to another element or molecule. When this happens, it creates an electrical current. In this ionic form, potassium is call and electrolyte.

Potassium in your body

There is only 3-4 oz. of potassium in your body at one time. But this small amount creates a body that can recover from disease or injuries quickly. It does this by using albumin, casein, and fibrin to repair and rebuild areas and to bring in more oxygen to the injured area.

Your body increases in efficiency when you have the excess potassium. Here are some of the benefits of potassium:

- Enzyme production
- Improves elimination of wastes

- Increases arterial and venous circulation
- Improves sexual function
- Improves heart function
- Improves nervous system and brain performance
- Controls cell life and function
- Alkalizes the blood and the body
- Maintains nerve electrical conduction
- Improves hair growth
- Active in skin health
- Promotes fibrin
- Controls muscle coordination
- Reduces internal oxidation
- Reduces pain
- Reduces intercellular edema
- Improves vigor and reduces low energy levels
- Reduces aches and pains

- Reduces anxiety

- Maintains heartbeat

Your body uses potassium to create normal body growth and function. It plays a key factor in maintaining heart and kidney function. Potassium is needed to utilize carbohydrates and to build proteins. Without potassium, your skin will become dehydrated and your skin will prematurely develop wrinkles.

Dehydrated or Dry Skin

If you suffer from dry skin, you need potassium. This mineral keeps your skin hydrated and moist from the inside. Taking a good potassium or eating more potassium foods will help to return your skin back to normal.

Potassium is also involved in new skin cell growth. Scars and blemishes will disappear sooner with good body levels of potassium. Without the proper levels, your skin will appear dull and cracked.

Improves hair Growth

When you have a lot of potassium in your body, your chances of going bald are less. Your roots are stronger and your hair stands are thicker. If you're a woman, your hair will grow longer and stronger.

There are many reasons why you might have hair loss. Stress, lack of minerals, lack of vitamins, pollution, poor hair care, use of bad hair product is some of the reasons for hair loss. But for sure, lack of potassium is also another reason. Start eating more potassium foods and you will see less hair loss.

Eating excess salt has an effect on hair growth. Salt interferes with the normal function of hair cell growth. Reducing the amount of salt you use in your food will help your hair growth. Use herbs and spices more in flavoring your food.

Controls muscle coordination

Strong, muscular, and athlete men have a

lot of potassium in their body. The high level of potassium gives them a strong nervous system, good nerve function, and brain activity. This occurs because potassium attracts oxygen. This excess oxygen gives these people the energy to perform all their athletic activities.

Your muscles need potassium for natural contraction and relaxation. It is needed for muscle tissue growth. A lack of potassium can result in tissue degradation.

A lack of blood potassium is called hypokalemia. This condition can cause heart muscle palpitations and many other conditions.

Muscle Cramps

You can have muscle cramps in the legs or anywhere in your body. Calcium and magnesium are necessary to eliminate or reduce cramps. In addition, potassium is also necessary to reduce or eliminate cramps.

Potassium is needed for smooth muscle functioning.

Improves elimination of wastes

When you have excess potassium the kidneys remove it from your blood. Potassium is also removed from your body through tears, perspiration, and fecal matter. Potassium is also used up in combining with phosphorous, chlorine, and sulfur.

When you lack potassium in the colon, the waste in the colon starts to ferment and putrefy and this feeds the bad bacteria and allows them to multiply. With the addition of body heat, this fermenting matter produces gases, toxins, and acids that get re-absorbed back into your bloodstream. The lack of potassium in your body will produce auto-intoxication and cause self-poisoning.

Cancer

In the case of cancer, it is important to keep high levels of potassium in the body with a reduced intake of table salt to prevent the formation of new tumors.

Fibrocystic Tumors

Fibrocystic tumors are made of potassium. When potassium is in balance in your body, your body will have normal function. Potassium has to be in balance with sodium, cesium, rubidium, iodine, and lithium.

Brain Growth

It is now known that the brain can grow new brain cells. But to do this, it needs that right nutrition and glucose. You can supplement with potassium to gain better brain function. Potassium helps to carry more oxygen to your brain, which helps to learn and to memorize.

Diabetes

If you have low levels of potassium, this can cause low blood sugar. For this reason, diabetics should continually eat high potassium foods and take supplements.

Alkaline Body

Perhaps, one of the main functions of potassium is in neutralizing body acids. It can help in making your body more alkaline. An alkaline body is a normal condition for your body. In an alkaline state, your body functions the way it should. More oxygen is routed to all parts of your body. Diseases do not function very good in an alkaline body full of oxygen.

To make your body alkaline, not only is more potassium need, but other minerals are also needed: sodium, magnesium, calcium, and D3. Check out my book called "Alkaline Body or Acid Body."

Making your body Alkaline should be one of your major goals in getting healthier. When you do this you will see a major change in your wellness.

3: How Potassium Prevents Diseases

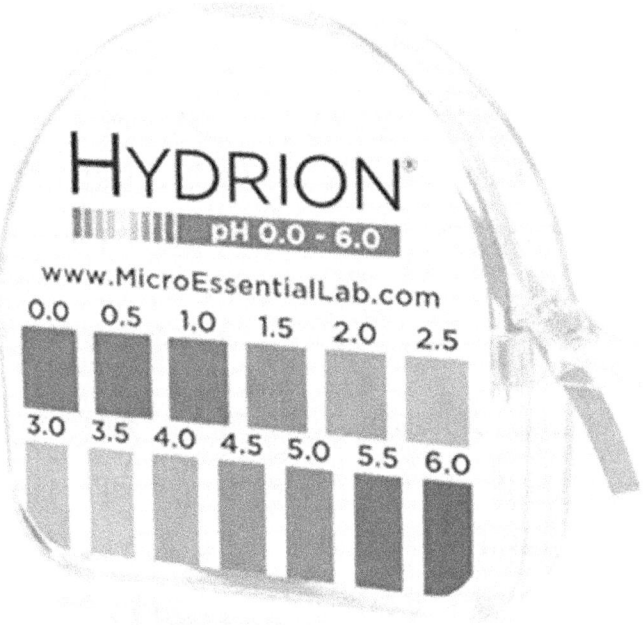

Alkalizes the blood and the body

Remember that the body's pH should be in the range of 7.2, which makes the body alkaline. Potassium is known for its ability to neutralize body acids and keep your body at 7.2 pH. In addition, Potassium and sodium chloride work in all areas of your body to neutralize acids and toxins. Potassium chloride is mostly found in your muscle tissues, red blood cells and nerve tissues where it neutralizes acids created during physical activities.

When the pH in the liquid outside your cells drops, potassium inside the cells comes out to bring the liquid pH back up to normal.

Acid Binding

There are certain minerals that are called acid binding. And these minerals found in fruits and vegetables are Sodium, potassium, chloride, calcium, phosphorus, magnesium.

What acid binding means is when you eat fruits with these minerals, they will seek out acids in your body and combine with them to neutralize them by creating a new chemical called alkaline forming ash.

Alkaline Ash

Now this alkaline forming ash has tied up

an acid and is now carried to the kidney where it is expelled as urine.

Different reactions can occur when an acid-binding mineral, like say potassium or sodium encounters an acid. Of course, acids in the body are toxic, so the body has the priority of getting rid of them fast since they can damage tissue and cause pain and disease.

So you can see the importance of getting a lot of alkaline minerals into your body. Without them, acids which do not get bonded to an alkaline mineral would move into body tissue and continue their body damage. Having an excess of acid in your body results in what is called an acid body. An acid body occurs when you don't have enough fruits and vegetables in your diet.

It is believed that cancer lives and thrives better in an acid body, which means a body liquid of 7.0 pH or lower. And, when your blood pH leans towards an acid condition, your nervous system and brain start to slow down.

The liquid is acidic when its pH is between 1.0 to 6.99 pH.

Potassium also works to:

- Reduce stomach acids
- Reduce intestinal acids
- Improve stomach, intestinal, and colon peristalsis
- Increases the alkalinity of cells, blood, lymph, body fluids and solids
- Improves heart action
- Improves Arterial pressure
- Stabilizes blood pressure and circulation
- Promotes good kidney action
- Calms the heart and nerves
- Prevents constipation and dehydration
- Improves the activity of the adrenal and pituitary glands

- Combines with albumin to form brain gray matter

Controls muscle coordination

When you use muscles as you do various activities, you produce monopotassium phosphate, lactic acid, and carbon dioxide. If you do not eliminate these acids, muscles will function properly. Potassium is necessary to eliminate these acids. Potassium salts such as potassium chloride and sodium chloride are necessary for your muscles structure so that glycogen can be converted to muscle energy so that you can have good muscle movement and strengthen.

Reduces pain

Potassium is a natural pain reducer which helps to control headaches, uterine pains, convulsions, and neuralgia. It helps to give you sound sleep and promotes nerve action. It helps you to reduce anxiety, stress, worry, fear, and grief. All sorts of issues related to over excitement are reduced by potassium, such as excess sexual excitement, hysterical convulsions, or uterine convulsions.

Excesses of potassium

When you have a slight excess of potassium in your diet or in your body, this is not a problem. It is quickly used up since it works through your whole body to provide you with powerful muscle action, mental capability, the calming action of the heart and mind, and powerful eyesight.

But when you have too much potassium, it has a weakening effect in your body. It has a paralytic effect on your autonomic nervous system, the motor and sensory nerves and brain functions. An excess of potassium causes a reduction in sodium and chlorine by causing their precipitation.

Excess potassium will cause thought confusion and weak reasoning and unfounded ideas. Imagination and creativity are dulled and memory becomes reduced. Excess blood moves to brain areas that cause wild and violent impulses.

You will see an increase in pulse rate, and blood pressure when you have excess potassium. You will have excess urination, perspiration, and muscle weakness.

Excess potassium attacks hemoglobin, causes vomiting, stomach pains, cramps, heart failure, coma, jaundice, convulsions, diarrhea, skin ulcers, tissue dryness, and skin pustules.

You can accumulate excess potassium when you eat preserved meats. Use drugs that contain potassium bromide, potassium phosphate, potassium carbonate, or potassium sulfate. If you eat a diet high in potassium or take an excess of potassium supplements you can also accumulate an excess of potassium in your body.

Having excess potassium in your body is not a common situation since the kidneys will remove excess potassium and excrete it. But when you have kidney malfunction this can lead to excess potassium, if you are eating a diet high in potassium or are taking potassium supplements. A deficiency in potassium is more typical, since most people may not eat foods high in potassium or take potassium supplements. And, on occasion, the kidney can excrete potassium even when you are low in body potassium.

Potassium deficiency

If you lack potassium in your body, you need to correct this condition right away. Blood tests and your doctor can help you determine if you have low blood potassium. Some of the symptoms of low-level potassium are:

- Appetite loss
- Muscle weakness and fatigue
- Muscle cramps
- Anemia
- A state of confusion and irritability
- Mild to severe constipation

- Excretion of calcium in urine

- Severe headaches

- Abnormal heartbeat

- High blood pressure

Improving Heart Function

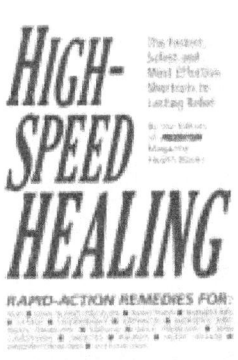

If potassium deficiency is not taken care of, your heart will become irregular, causing a decrease in the blood being pumped into your body. This condition can lead to a stroke or heart attack.

In their book, High-Speed Healing, Editors of Prevention Magazine Health Books, 1991, Pennsylvania, reported that,

"Potassium-rich foods have been shown to lower blood pressure, and a deficiency of potassium - whose chemical symbol is K – has been linked to an increase in blood pressure. Fresh fruits and vegetables – especially bananas and potatoes – dry beans, and whole grains are rich in potassium, says potassium expert George, Webb, Ph. D., an associate professor of Physiology and Biophysics at the University of Vermont Medical College. In one study, 859 people over a 12 year period reduced their risk of dying from stroke by 40 percent by eating just one extra serving of fresh fruits or vegetables a day. And the more of the potassium-rich foods they ate, the lower their risk."

The reason high blood pressure is controlled by potassium is that it has the ability to restore normal kidney function. The kidneys play an important function in blood pressure.

If you are on are on any type of diuretic medication, you will tend to lose potassium. If you have a severe case of diarrhea or long-standing diarrhea, you will also be losing potassium that your body needs.

Potassium is one of the superstars for lowering high blood pressure and cholesterol.

In other studies, it was shown that some men, after a year on a high potassium diet, could reduce their high blood medication by 50%. And, other men, in the study, were able to stop their drug medication completely. This was done by having 3 to 6 servings of high-potassium foods every day.

Stroke

In her book called, Food Your Miracle Medicine, Jean Carpet, Harper Collins Publishers, 1993, reports on this study,

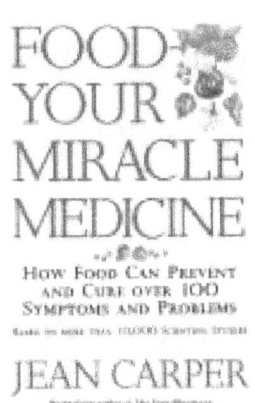

"Eat just one extra serving of a potassium-rich food every day; that too may reduce your risk of stroke by 40 percent. That's what researchers discovered by analyzing the diets of a group of 859 men and women over age 50, living in southern California. The investigators documented that small differences of potassium in the diet predicted who would die of a stroke twelve years later.

Remarkably, nobody with the highest intake of potassium, more than 3,500 mg a day, died of a stroke. However, those who regularly ate the least potassium, less than 1950 mg, per day had much higher fatal stroke rates than all the others. Among those who skimped the most on potassium, the odds of stroke deaths shot up 2.6 times in men and 4.8 times in women. Further, the more potassium-rich foods the subjects ate, generally, the fewer strokes they had. Indeed, the researchers concluded that with every extra daily 400 mg of potassium in the food, the odds of a fatal stroke dropped 40 percent."

Alcoholics

People who are alcoholics have poor diets, are anorexic tend to be deficient in potassium. If you are on a diuretic drug, you will lose potassium and eating potassium foods will be of no value since the will be excreted.

Respiratory Illness

When you have too much salt in your diet, you get your potassium-sodium ratio out of balance. This will affect your nervous system. Since your nervous system controls your respiratory system, this can lead to a variety of respiratory illness such as emphysema or bronchitis.

Potassium obtained from vegetable soups, fruits, or supplements has a laxative effect in the colon.

Kidney Stones

In Blended Medicine, Michael Castleman, Rodale, 2000, says that,

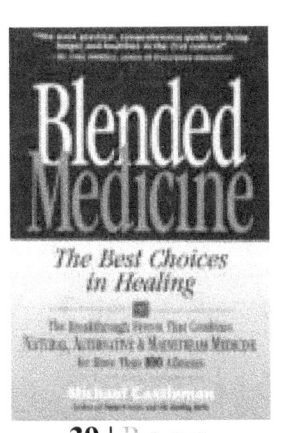

"At the Kaiser Permanente Medical Care Program in Oakland, California, Brue, Ettinger, M.D., gave 64 people with recurrent kidney stones either a supplement containing potassium and magnesium

citrate or a placebo.   After 3 years, the supplement takers had 85 percent fewer recurrences than the placebo takers.

For her patients, clinical nutritionist Shari Lieberman Ph.D. prescribes 200 milligrams of potassium and 500 milligrams of magnesium every day. Because of potentially serious risks associated with potassium, take supplements only under your doctor's care."

Muscle Cramping

When you exercise or do some activity that you typically don't do, your muscles can become sore or cramp. This can occur when you don't have enough minerals to neutralize the lactic acid that is created during your exercise.

When you develop this kind of soreness, you can take a supplement of potassium with calcium and magnesium. A better way to get the potassium you need is to eat potassium-rich food and then add your calcium magnesium capsules.

In Prevention Magazine's Complete Book Of Vitamins and Minerals, Rodale Press, 1988, they say that,

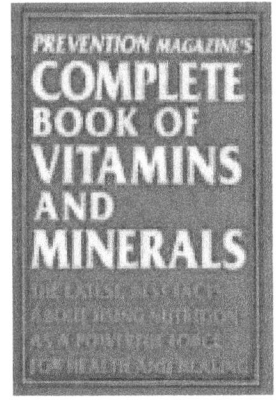

"There is far from a consensus on the effects of mineral loss in exercise, but add a few more to the list of nutrients to monitor. Potassium, magnesium, and zinc are lost in sweat, though losses vary widely from one person to the other.

A nutrition expert and a runner himself, Gabe Mirkin, M.D., coauthor of the Sports Medicine Book, says exercisers who feel weak and tired maybe suffering from 'the mineral blues,' a deficiency of potassium and magnesium inside muscle cells. When Dr. Mirkin, who ran 100 miles a month, suddenly found that running a quarter-mile 'felt like a marathon,' he had his blood tested. He learned that he was potassium deficient, something he remedied with copious quantities of fruit juices."

Diabetics

Potassium assists iodine in creating thyroid hormones, which increase the metabolism and regulate the metabolism of glucose.

Constipation

Because potassium is involved in muscle contractions and function, the lack of potassium can lead to constipation. The severity of the reduced peristaltic colon action will depend on the deficiency in potassium and the length of this deficiency.

In Hidden Secrets of Super Perfect Health At Any Age Book II, William L. Fischer, Fischer Publishing Corporation, Ohio, 1986, writes,

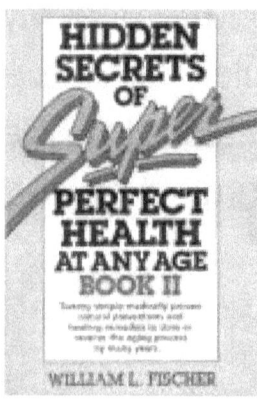

"Persons on a refined, denatured diet deficient in potassium quickly develop fatigue, listlessness, gas pains, constipation, insomnia and low

blood sugar. Muscles become soft and flabby and the pulse becomes slow week and irregular. By far the greatest harm caused by a lack of potassium is the effect on the heart. Heart attacks are often associated with a low potassium intake. An excessive intake of sodium, salt, can produce a potassium deficiency even when it appears the diet is adequately supplied. Yeast is an incomparable source of needed potassium. "

4: Foods high in potassium

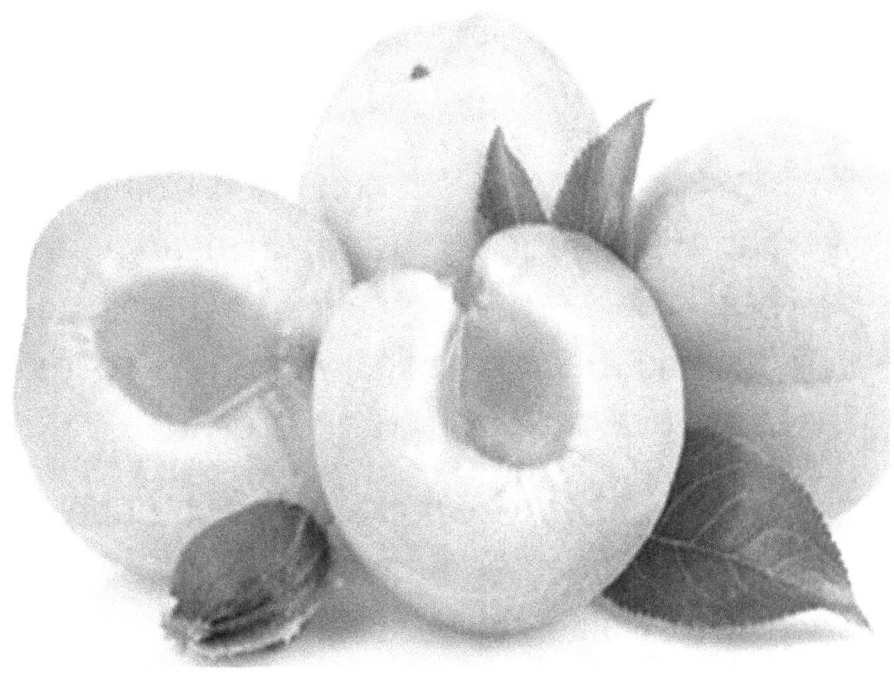

One reason you may be low in potassium is that when you boil vegetables you lose potassium into the water or it's lost with the steam. Of course, one way to minimize this loss is to also drink the liquid you use in boiling.

Potassium Cocktail

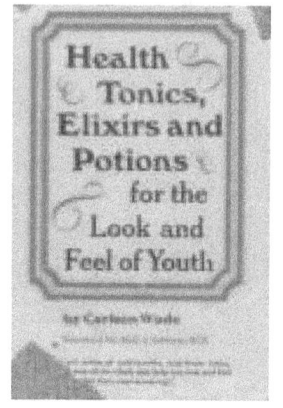

This works out ok when you make a soup or when you create a potassium cocktail as outlined in Health Tonics, Elixirs, and Potions, Carlson Wade, 1971, New York,

"Select sun-dried fruits such as apricots, prunes, raisins, pears, and peaches. Be sure to obtain sun-dried fruits that have not been chemically dried or treated. These are available at health stores.

Heat a kettle of water. After it bubbles, turn off the heat and let the water simmer down. Next place an assortment of sun-dried fruits in a deep bowl. Cover with the simmered water. Place a cover on the bowl. Let it remain at room temperature overnight. In the morning pour off one or two cups of the juice and drink. This is your Potassium Cocktail. You may eat the fruit for breakfast. This Potassium Cocktail has a power-packed mineral benefit that is reportedly second to none for its effectiveness in rejuvenating the bloodstream and recreating the sought-after look and feel of youth."

Potassium Broth

Here is another way to create a highly concentrated drink or liquid of potassium. These cocktails or broths are a fantastic way to get back into balance when you lack potassium and are trying to get back to normal from a major illness. They not only provide you with potassium but with an array of minerals that helps you clean out your intestinal tract and to rejuvenate your blood.

In her book, The Body-Smart System, Helene, Silver, Bantam Books, 1990, outline a broth that you can create to use as stock broth or as a full meal. To do this, you need to do the following:

Gather these vegetables,

14, carrots with tops, 14 celery stalks with

tops, 2 bunches of beet tops, 4 potatoes, 2 onions, 4 cloves of garlic, 3 summer squash, 3 zucchini, 2 handfuls of parsley

Place all chopped vegetables in a pot and cover with clean water, place a cover over the pot, boil and simmer for 30 minutes. After, turn the heat off and allow to stand for another 30 minutes.

Remove the green tops from the vegetables and get rid of them. Put the remaining vegetables into a blender, but add a little of the clear broth, 1/4 cup, into the blender to puree them.

Now you can use the pureed vegetables as a meal and the clear broth as stock broth for other soups.

You can refrigerate the unused parts and hold for up to 4 days.

Foods High In Potassium

The foods highest in potassium are sun-dried black olives, potato peel broth, dulse, kelp, bitter greens, Irish moss. Other foods high in potassium are:

Almonds	kale	spinach
Anise seeds	lentil	lima beans
Apples	parsley	dried pears
Bananas	beans	beets greens
Black cherries	pecans	raisins
Broccoli	rice bran	carrots
Sesame seeds	cashews	cucumbers
Dates	turnips	fish
Grapes	watercress	wheat germ
Wheat bran	tomatoes	yams
Berries	oranges	garlic
Blackstrap Molasses		natural honey
Avocados	dried apricots	pineapples
Sardines	`	winter squash prunes
Cantaloupe	sweet potato	yeast
Coconut water,	Pomegranate	

Bananas

In his book, Arthritis Rx, Vijay Vad, M.D., Gotham Books, 2006, talks about bananas,

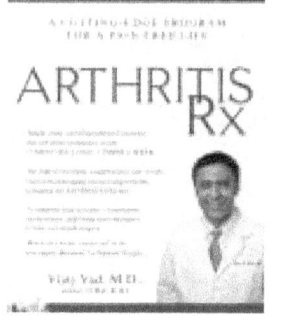

"Bananas are high in vitamin B6, potassium, and iron. The FDA has endorsed the value of potassium: 'Diets containing foods that are good sources of potassium and low in sodium may reduce the risk of high blood pressure and stroke.' One study of 40,000 American male health professionals over four years determined that men who ate diets higher in potassium had a substantially reduced risk of stroke. They [bananas] also help with weight loss because they are rich in fiber, low in fat, and quite filling, and they feed the natural acidophilus bacteria in the intestines, necessary for proper digestion. What more could you ask from a delicious fruit that comes in its own wrapper?"

Yogurt

Plain yogurt is better nutritionally then milk. Eight ounces contains up to 40% of your daily calcium requirements. If you can't tolerate milk, you should be able to eat yogurt without any digestive problems.

Yogurt contains protein, calcium, potassium, phosphorus, vitamin B6, B12, niacin, and folic acid and is known to have just as much potassium as a banana.

Chose the yogurt that is labeled "sugar-free, contains active, cultures, and/or plain yogurt." Remember that when yogurt is heat treated is loses most of its health benefits, since heat kills the beneficial bacteria.

Potassium and sodium balance

When thinking about potassium, you need to think about potassium and sodium balance. Potassium does not work independently in your body and must be brought into your body in food that is balanced with sodium. This balance is only found in raw, unpreserved fruits and vegetables. In your body, a specific ratio of potassium and sodium must be maintained so that you can have the best health.

Most produce has 20 times more potassium than sodium. In your body, it has 3 times more potassium than sodium.

Your body finds it easy to excrete potassium since it comes out of your urine, sweat, fecal matter, tears, and in all other types of body secretions. However, your body tends to hold on to sodium, so if you have an excess of sodium this will affect your potassium-sodium balance. Most fruits and vegetables are low in sodium and in a natural diet containing raw fruits and vegetables, the body would be low in sodium and that is why it holds on to sodium. But when eating processed foods, which are high in sodium, your body ends up having high sodium content, thereby changing the potassium – sodium ratio, which leads to disease.

Your kidney will excrete 10 mg of sodium, if you are low in sodium, but will excrete up to 240 mg of potassium, since normally you have more potassium than sodium in your body.

You will notice that most processed food have high sodium content. Salt is used as a preservative and helps to inhibit molds and bacteria and to help food keep its color. The use of salt is saving manufacturer tremendous money while causing you untold bad health. Eating these foods will create an imbalance in your potassium to sodium ratio. Slight good changes in what you eat and the way you eat will improve your body's potassium – sodium balance.

Here is a small list of foods that are out of balance and contain from 2 to 10 times more sodium than potassium, the reverse of what it should be:

Apple pie

white bread   cheese spreads

Cheese   cottage cheese

Dry cereal	frankfurters
green olives	cold cuts
Pancakes	peanut butter
canned peas	canned salmon
Potato chips	Ritz crackers
Saltines sauerkraut	canned tuna

Reduce your salt intake by using herbs to season your food. Always look at the content of the food you buy. Buy more those foods that don't have added salt. Instead of salt on your eggs try using coriander, parsley, tarragon, thyme, or basil. Use herbs to season your chicken or fish.

Try to get more potassium into your diet than you do salt. Use raw fruits and vegetables. You can cook vegetables slightly and still maintain a good ratio. Eat raw nuts. Best nuts to eat are almonds, pecans, and pine.

Here is a list of good foods and the milligram amount of potassium they have in **100 gram.**

Dulse	8060
Kelp	5273
Irish moss	2844
Pistachio nuts	972
Dehydrated prunes	940
Sunflower seeds	**920**
Dried lentils	790
Raisins	763
Parsley	694
Avocado	604
Yams	600
Spinach	470
Potato with skin	407
Banana	370
Carrots	340

Potassium in one cup (mg)

White beans	3636
Dried apricots	1511
Beet greens	1309
Prunes	1274
Avocado	975
Acorn Squash	431
Pomegranate	282
Coconut water	240
Carrot juices	236
Yogurt	227
Salmon (half a fillet)	198
Spinach	167
One Lg Banana	136
Sweet potatoes	133
Swiss chard	36

Here is a list of foods or body conditions that will deplete your stored body potassium:

Alcohol antibiotics diarrhea

Caffeine diuretics

Sweating high cholesterol

Cortisone aldosterone

Pain and inflammation products

Laxatives salt

Stress sugar

5: Using potassium supplements

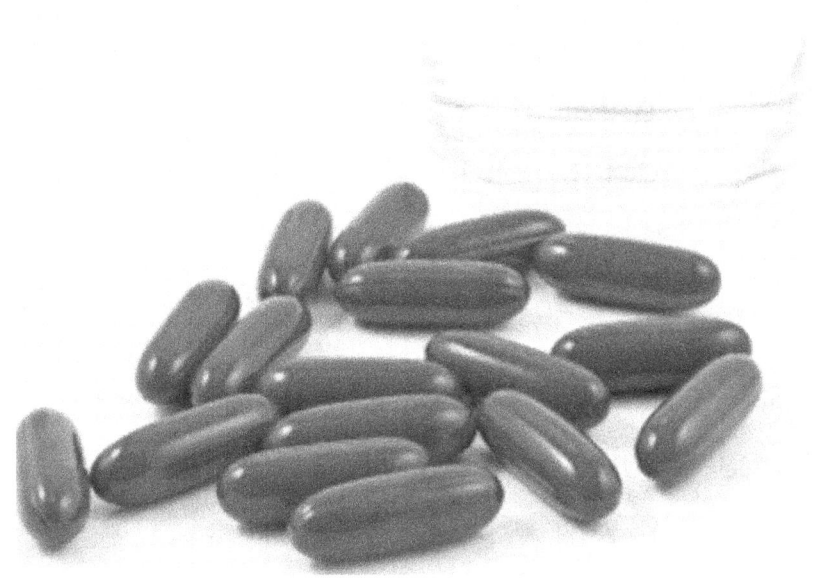

Potassium supplements may be prescribed by your doctor when you have chronic diarrhea, excess vomiting, high blood pressure, overuse of laxatives, or diabetic acidosis.

Take caution when using potassium supplements, since there are dangers with overdosing. If you are on medication or are not in good health, then it is best to see a doctor before taking potassium supplements.

Use food first to get more potassium. Food is very high in potassium and you can easily increase your intake of potassium to 5000mg by picking the right foods. Typically you may want to only increase your potassium to around 3000mg for general maintenance.

When using potassium supplements always take them with meals. Potassium requires other minerals and vitamins to be present for adequate digestion and adsorption. The actual form you use is important so that your body will be able to absorb it.

If you feel you are low in potassium it is a good idea to ask your doctor for a nutritional blood test for potassium and other minerals. In this way, you know for sure if you are low and need to work on this part of your nutritional health.

When you are on a diuretic, you deplete

your potassium, so it's a good idea to add a potassium supplement to your diet. Take this supplement with your meals so that it can mix with the other vitamins and minerals you have eaten.

Potassium glycerophosphate – is one of best forms of potassium, since it is easily and quickly absorbed by your body and cell walls.

Potassium citrate – is readily absorbed and it is useful in restoring urinary citrate back to normal. Citrate is important because it reduces the formation of calcium salt stones. In the urine, citrate can be reduced when you eat excess sodium and protein. In addition, Potassium citrate reduces urinary calcium excretion, which helps lessen the loss of calcium.

Potassium Aspartate – is a form where potassium is tied to the aspartic acid, which is an acidic amino acid. When minerals are tied to amino acids they pass easily and quickly through your intestinal wall and into your bloodstream.

Potassium Chlorine - is a salt substitute and may be found in some supplements. It is not a good idea to use potassium chlorine in place of sodium chlorine, table salt since after potassium is used up the chlorine can combine sodium and thereby reducing the sodium available to work with potassium in the Potassium Sodium Pump. Also, Potassium Chlorine interferes with the absorption of vitamin B12.

When taking potassium supplements, make sure the formulation also has magnesium. Magnesium is necessary to maintain potassium in the body. Also, your heart muscle will not hold potassium without the presence of magnesium.

Final Comments

Potassium works with sodium to create the Potassium-Sodium Pump that allows nutrients to enter each cell. The Pump also allows toxins and other waste to exit the cell. When the body is low in calcium, calcium is pulled out of storage from the cell interior and out into the body where it is needed.

When you are deficient in potassium you will experience body weakness and tiredness. Your mental abilities will diminish and the nervous system will suffer from reduced nerve transmissions.

Building up excess potassium in the body has similar effects as not having enough. It is best to add those raw foods that have the proper potassium to sodium ratio, especially if you have a diet high in processed foods. Using potassium supplement must be done with caution. If you do use them, use low doses so you can see the results. You can take your saliva pH and then measure it again after a week of supplements to check your progress.

Things for you to do

Look at the list of foods high in potassium and add at least 3 to 4 of them to your daily or weekly diet. As usual, check your saliva pH and then do it again after a week of using more potassium foods.

To get more potassium in your diet you can take from 100mg to 500mg per day. The higher dose is for when you are dealing with high blood pressure or other illnesses. Just to increase your potassium intake, use 100 - 200mg per day.

About The Author And Other Resources

Rudy Silva is a natural consultant nutritionist educated in the United State of Nutrition and Physics.   He is a graduate of the San Jose State University in California. He is the author of 30 other e-books on natural remedies.   He has authored a newsletter in natural remedies for over 4 years.   He has many websites promoting special recommended products and information.

Resource page

Other books written by this author can be found by going to the internet and using the keyword, Rudy Silva Books.

If you need support or want to promote any of his books, please contact him at rss41@yahoo.com and expect a reply within 24 hours.   He looks forward to hearing from you and is happy to help you understand his material on natural and nutritional health.

Give A Review

And, don't forget to give a review for this book so that others can gain the benefits of what is in this e-book.

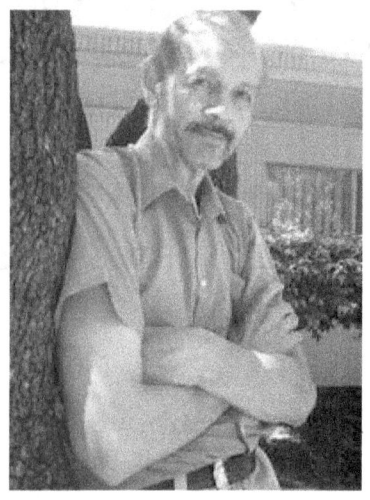

To you, for creating better health and more happiness in your life,

Rudy S Silva

www.ingramcontent.com/pod-product-compliance
Lightning Source LLC
Chambersburg PA
CBHW070818290526
45795CB00002B/748